HOW TO TREAT HAIR LOSS NATURALLY AS FAST AS POSSIBLE

How To Treat Hair Loss, How To Treat Hair Loss Fast, How To Treat Hair Loss Naturally Fast, How To Treat Hair Loss For Women

Okesanjo A.A

CHAPTER ONE
Introduction

Please read this book carefully from start to the end if you are truly prepared to do what it takes to regrow your hair. If you're not prepared to take some extreme action that will actually get results, this might not be for you. In this book I provide detailed instructions on how to perform at-home.

In this book I provide detailed instructions on how to perform at-home procedures that eliminate each of the key causes of hair loss. These procedures have been refined over many years, to produce the ultimate hair growth methodology. This can all be done at home, on your own, with the use of a few inexpensive, safe products.

Hair loss is not a simple problem. It is extremely difficult to reverse — you must understand that if you want to start regrowing your hair. If you truly want to start regrowing your hair you have to do some fairly extreme things.

Buying some hair loss supplements and taking them every day, or some Minoxidil and using it every day is just not going to do it. You'll do nothing more than waste your money for a few years and then one day you'll realize that what I'm saying is right. Those hair loss products don't work.

If you want to stop your hair loss and regrow your hair you need to intensely feed your hair. Not just feed it a little bit. *You need to feed it a lot.*

The truth about hair loss revealed

The same thing is happening to millions of people worldwide, yet they do nothing about it. The truth is very simple. The truth about hair loss is this, you can't regrow your hair if your hair is not receiving the nutrients it needs to grow.

That is a very simple and obvious statement I know, but keep reading because it's very important you understand this if you want to regrow your hair, make it thicker, shinier, longer and healthier.

Your hair receives nutrients from your blood. Tiny blood vessels connect to your hair in your scalp. As we age, some peoples' scalps change and the blood supply to the hair follicles becomes restricted. It can get so restricted that the follicles receive no nutrients at all and they become completely dormant.

Early signs that this has started happening are unhealthy looking hair. Then the hair begins to thin. Then noticeable hair loss becomes apparent. Hair loss is extremely common, affecting about 50 million men and 30 million women in the U.S. alone, not to talk of other countries.

About 50% of men will have some hair loss by the time they turn 50. Hair loss is not life-threatening, though it can have devastating psychological effects, particularly in women.

CHAPTER TWO
What Are Causes of Hair Loss?

Hair loss is often caused by genetics, that is, it runs in families. In general, it is not a symptom of disease, however, thyroid disease, anemia, ringworm of the scalp, and anorexia can cause hair loss. In addition, some medications such as cancer chemotherapy may cause temporary hair loss.

Hair growth usually returns to normal when the medications are stopped. In some cases, hormones changes after giving birth or during menopause can cause thinning hair.

CHAPTER THREE
Types of Hair Loss

There are several types of hair loss, often classified by whether the loss is localized, or if it affects large areas, or if the hair loss is patchy or affects the entire scalp. Some of the more common hair loss causes are discussed below.

Well, we need to make one thing very clear: not all hair loss can be treated!

Essentially, there are three basic kinds of hair loss:

- Trauma-related hair loss - If you suffer physical, mental, or emotional trauma, it may "shock" your hair from the active growth phase to the shedding phase. Many people lose hair after a car accident, loss of a loved one, or pregnancy, all because of the trauma.

  Thankfully, this is a hair loss because that clears up on its own. Your hair will usually grow back in time.

- Hormone or disorder-related hair loss - If you are suffering hair loss as a result of a hormonal imbalance (excessive androgen leading to male and female pattern baldness) or a disorder that causes hair loss (autoimmune conditions where your body treats your hairs and follicles like invaders), you need to look into medical options for treating the hair loss.

In many cases, the hair loss can only be slowed, not stopped or prevented completely. Consult your doctor to find out more.

- Other causes of hair loss - If your hair is falling out as a result of insufficient protein, vitamin, or mineral intake, the good news is that you can do something about it! The same goes for hair loss caused by poor circulation, poor scalp health, excessive free radical activity in your body, and other causes not related to either of the two listed above.

We've come up with a lot of solutions on how to treat hair loss quickly, but they're all for the "other causes of hair loss". They all focus on improving the health of your hair, scalp, circulatory system, and body overall, ensuring that your body has everything it needs to create new, healthy hair on its own.

With no further ado, here are our tips to help you know how to treat hair loss quickly the natural way in the next chapter.

CHAPTER FOUR
Treatments

Eat Right

The food you eat can have a HUGE effect on your hair health!

Think of your hair (and skin) as your body's best ways of telling you what's going on inside you. If things inside your body are off balance, your hair and skin will suffer. If things inside your body are healthy, you'll have strong, lustrous, and healthy hair.

If your hair is falling out, it may be a very clear sign that you're not getting enough of certain vitamins, minerals, antioxidants, fatty acids, or amino acids. Eating more of "the right" foods will help to improve the health of your hair.

So, what are these "right" foods? Here is a list of foods that will make your hair stronger, longer, and less likely to fall out:

- Salmon - Salmon, and all fatty fish, contain Omega-3 fatty acids. These fatty acids improve circulation, reduce inflammation, and strengthen your heart muscles. They also protect your skin and scalp from infection. The high-fat content of fish will add a beautiful luster to your hair.

- Guava - Did you know that a single guava contains all the Vitamin C you need to consume in a single day? Add two or three of these bad boys to your daily diet, and the influx of Vitamin C will enhance the protection of your hair. This vitamin can reduce the risk of breakage and split ends.

- Yogurt - If you want healthy hair, you need a lot of protein. Hair is made up of a protein called keratin, which can only be produced if you have enough amino acids. Thankfully, yogurt (particularly Greek yogurt) is an amazing source of protein, one that will help your hair to grow faster.

  It also contains Vitamin B5, which reduces hair thinning and hair loss.

- Spinach - Spinach is loaded with healthy nutrients, including Vitamin A, Vitamin C, folic acid, iron, and polyphenols. All of these nutrients contribute to making your hair healthier, and they will keep your hair moisturized–thus protected from drying out and becoming brittle.

  All dark, leafy greens are good for your hair.

- Sweet Potatoes - Sweet potatoes are rich in beta-carotene, an antioxidant that your body turns into Vitamin A. Beta carotene can help to reduce free radical activity and oxidative stress in your body, improve circulation, and protect your hair from drying out.

The vitamin also encourages the sebaceous glands in your scalp to produce more sebum, the skin oil that coats your hair and skin to protect it.

- Red Meat — Red meat isn't just a good source of protein and metabolism-boosting B vitamins, it's also one of the best sources of iron. A lack of iron can lead to hair loss, as your body needs iron to produce the red blood cells that bring oxygen and nutrient throughout your body.

  If there is a shortage of red blood cells, your skin and hair are the first to suffer. By eating more red meat, you give your body more iron, thus ensuring you have all the red blood cells needed to keep your hair and skin healthy– along with the rest of your body, of course!

- Avocadoes — Avocadoes are packed with Vitamin E, which acts as a protective coating to keep moisture locked inside your hair and skin. Without enough Vitamin E, there's a risk of your hair and scalp drying out. When your hair and scalp get too dry, the hair gets brittle and tends to break.

The fatty acids in avocados will also improve your circulation and keep your heart sending oxygen and nutrients to your head.

- Chicken — Poultry is a lean meat, meaning it's rich in protein but without as much fat as other proteins. Protein helps to keep your hair in the "growing" phase for longer, and a lack of protein causes your hair to enter the "resting" phase.

  If you want to encourage hair growth and increase the production of new hair cells, you definitely want more protein in your life. Chicken happens to be one of the best proteins around.

- Cinnamon — There are very few foods as effective at boosting circulation as cinnamon! It contains compounds that dilate your blood vessels, increasing the flow of blood throughout your body. The more your blood flows, the more oxygen and nutrients reach your scalp and hair–ergo, the healthier they are!

- Oysters — If you want to have healthy hair, you need more zinc. Zinc plays a role in your immune health, but it also plays a role in the production of new hair. Without zinc, your body can't produce new hair cells. By getting more zinc, you ensure a steady production of hair cells, leading to longer and stronger hair.

- Eggs — Yet another great source of protein, eggs are also packed with B vitamins, iron, and other vital nutrients. But it's biotin, a B vitamin, that makes eggs truly awesome for your hair. A biotin deficiency can lead to hair loss, so it's vital that you get more of this important nutrient in your diet.

  Few foods contain as much biotin as eggs. Plus, few foods are as delicious!

These are the main foods to eat if you want to know how to treat hair loss quickly, but there are so much more! Basically, if you want to have healthier hair, you need to follow a healthy diet. That means:

- Lots of fruits, veggies, nuts, seeds, and lean proteins

- Some complex carbs (whole grains) and animal fats

- Minimal sugar, caffeine, and alcohol consumption

- NO soda, heavily fried foods, or junk food

Follow this basic diet, and you'll have much healthier hair as a result!

Massage Your Scalp

Did you know that poor circulation of blood can cause hair loss? Think about it: your blood brings oxygen and nutrients, so if there's not enough blood flowing to your head, you're not getting enough nutrients.

Scalp massage is one of the best ways to increase blood flow to your scalp. The massage stimulates the capillaries beneath the skin, and the influx of blood will deliver a steady stream of nutrients to nourish your hair.

How do you massage your scalp? Easy: do it while in the shower!

Let warm water run over your hair, and use your fingers to massage your scalp gently. If you're applying shampoo or conditioner, even better. The massage will help to stimulate the flow of blood AND ensure the nutrients from the shampoo/conditioner penetrate your hair and scalp more effectively.

A few minutes of scalp massage every day can do wonders for your hair health

Control Stress

Stress is a killer! It won't just shorten your life and increase your risk of health problems, but it will kill off your hair.

When you're stressed, your body produces a lot of cortisol. This hormone keeps your body in "fight or flight" mode long after it should have returned to normal. It can also lead to hormonal imbalances that may contribute to your hair loss.

There's no way to avoid stress completely, but you do need to find ways to cope with it. Try these methods:

- Every hour, take 2 minutes to sit in silence with your eyes closed and just focus on your breathing.

- Every hour or so, take a short walk around the office to give your mind and body a break.

- Take time off on the weekends, and disconnect from everything and everyone.

- Find activities that you enjoy, and which help you to relax.

The more you fight stress, the healthier and happier you'll be!

Other Unique Remedies to Try

Here are a few more awesome remedies to try:

- Make a paste of 1 tablespoon of ground licorice root and 1 cup of milk. Apply it to the patches of thinning hair, let it sit overnight, and rinse in the morning. Licorice root is excellent for opening your pores, reducing irritation and inflammation, and soothing your scalp.

- Use aloe vera to promote hair growth. The alkalizing enzymes in aloe vera will restore your scalp to a healthier pH, reduce itching and dandruff, and add strength to your hair.

- Use onion juice. It may be stinky, but the high sulfur content of the juice will improve circulation to your scalp. Grate the onion, strain it to extract the juice, apply it to your hair, and let it sit for 30 minutes.

- Give your scalp an oil massage, using tea tree oil (diluted to 5%), almond oil, coconut oil, or essential oils. The oil will protect and nourish your hair and scalp, and the massage will stimulate blood flow.

- Use Indian gooseberry, or amla. Mix amla paste with coconut oil, and use it to massage your scalp. The combination is highly effective!

- Mix 1 egg with a tablespoon of honey, and apply it to the patches of thinning hair. Honey is a potent antibacterial (anti-dandruff) agent, and eggs are loaded with vital nutrients.

- Ultimate Solution: Visit Your Doctor

If you're not sure what's causing the hair loss, it may be a good idea to visit your doctor. The underlying cause may be nutrition-related, or it could have something to do with your hormone levels. Talk to your physician to find out if there is a hormone-based cause behind your hair loss, and take steps to deal with the problem before you really start losing hair!

CHAPTER FIVE
Women vs Men Hair

Is hair loss in women different from men?

Female-Pattern Baldness

Women lose hair on an inherited (genetic) basis, too, but female pattern hair loss tends to be more diffuse, with less likelihood of the crown and frontal hairline being lost. Although some women may notice hair thinning as early as their 20s, the pace of hair loss tends to be gradual, often taking years to become obvious to others.

There seems to be a normal physiologic thinning that comes with age and occurs in many women in their early to mid-30s. More women have underlying causes of hair loss than men. These include treatable conditions like anaemia and thyroid disease and polycystic ovary syndrome (PCOS).

These conditions are diagnosed by blood tests along with a historical and physical evidence. Although a few studies have suggested that baldness may be inherited through the mother's family genes, these theories require further testing.

Current studies are inconclusive. Although not indicated for female pattern balding spironolactone (Aldactone) has had some success in treating this condition.

While stories about hats choking off follicles or long hair pulling on the roots may be more folklore, repeat hair trauma like tightly woven hair pulled back and consistent friction can potentially worsen or cause localized hair loss in some individuals. Individuals who pull their hair tightly back in a rubber band can develop a localized hair loss at the front of the scalp.

Hair loss "myths" of special concern to women

- *Longer hair does not necessarily put a strain on roots.*

- *Shampooing does not accelerate hair loss*; it just removes those that were ready to fall out anyway.

- *Coloring, perming, and conditioning the hair do not usually cause hair loss.* Burns or severe processing may produce hair fragility and breakage. Styles that pull tight may cause some loss, but hair coloring and "chemicals" usually don't.

Male - Pattern Baldness

Androgenetic alopecia, also sometimes referred to as "male pattern baldness," accounts for the majority of hair loss in men, but it can also affect women. It is usually caused by a combination of hormones and genetics.

Some men may start to notice thinning hair as early as their 20s, and by age 50, 50% of men see some hair loss. Hair is usually lost in a pattern, starting at the temples, revealing the classic "M" shaped hairline seen as men age.

Myths About Male-Pattern Baldness

There are many myths about male-pattern baldness.

- MYTH: Baldness is inherited through the mother's side of the family. If your maternal grandfather was bald, you will be too.

- FACT: Genes for baldness can come from either parent.

- MYTH: Wearing hats strains hair follicles and causes hair loss.

- FACT: Unless your hat is so tight it cuts off circulation to hair follicles, it will not cause hair loss.

- MYTH: Using a blow dryer causes hair loss.

- FACT: Use of a blow dryer does not cause hair to fall out. However, frequent over-use of a hot dryer can cause hair to become brittle, damaged, and break, which may cause hair to appear thinner.

- MYTH: Washing hair too frequently or using certain styling products can cause hair to fall out.

- FACT: Shampoo and hair care products do not cause hair loss.

- MYTH: Massaging the scalp will help hair regrow by stimulating circulation around the follicles.

- FACT: It may make you feel good, but no studies have shown scalp massage helps regrow hair.

CHAPTER SIX
Pregnancy Hair Loss

What about pregnancy hair loss?

Pregnancy may cause many changes in the scalp hair. As the hormones fluctuate during pregnancy, a large number of women feel their hair thickens and becomes fuller. This may be related to change in the number of hairs cycling in the growth phase of hair growth, but the exact reason is unknown.

Quite often, there may be a loss of hair (telogen effluvium) after delivery or a few months later which will eventually normalize.

Female hair loss treatments

Include minoxidil (Rogaine), hair transplants, hair-powder fibers like Toppik, wigs, hair extensions, and weaves.

- Minoxidil (Rogaine) is available over the counter and available in 2%, 4%, and 5% concentrations. It may be something of a nuisance to apply twice daily, but it has been shown to help conserve hair and may even grow some. Minoxidil tends to grow very fine small hairs wherever it is applied.

It is important to avoid running the liquid onto the face or neck where it can also grow hair. It is marketed for women at the 2% concentration but may be used in higher strengths as directed by a doctor.

- Surgical procedures like hair transplants can be useful for some women as well as men to "fill in" thinned-out areas.

CHAPTER SEVEN
Home Remedies

What vitamins are good for hair loss?

Are there home remedies for hair loss?

These are the additional treatment to the ones raised above under chapter meant for Treatments.

A good daily multivitamin containing zinc, vitamin B, folate, iron, and calcium is a reasonable choice, although there is no good evidence that vitamins have any meaningful benefit in alopecia. Newer studies suggest that vitamin D may be somewhat helpful and worth considering.

Specific vitamin and mineral deficiencies like iron or vitamin B12 may be diagnosed by blood tests and treated.

Multiple vitamins, including BIOTIN, have been promoted for hair growth, but solid scientific studies for many of these claims are lacking. While taking biotin and other supplements marketed for hair, skin, and nails probably won't worsen anything, it may also not necessarily help the situation.

Therefore, advertised hair-
regrowth supplements should be approached with mild caution. There is only anecdotal evidence that oral or topical application garlic, onion juice, saw

palmetto, coconut oil, evening primrose oil, apple cider vinegar, creatine, and pumpkin seed oil are of benefit for hair loss.

CHAPTER EIGHT
How to Loss Hair

Can itchy scalp cause hair loss?

Itchy scalp may be a symptom of a scalp disease that could produce hair loss. Causes may include seborrheic dermatitis (dandruff) and psoriasis. Treatments may include medicated shampoos like ketoconazole (Nizoral), OTC dandruff shampoos, and topical steroid creams and lotions to help decrease itching.

What is the prognosis for hair loss?

The prognosis for androgenic non-scarring hair loss is guarded due to the fact that there is no cure for the problem. Medications must be taken indefinitely. Other types of hair loss have a good chance of spontaneously resolving.

CHAPTER NINE
How to Prevent Hair Loss

How do people prevent hair loss?

Hair-loss prevention depends on the underlying cause. Good hair hygiene with regular shampooing is a basic step but is probably of little benefit.
Good nutrition, especially adequate levels of iron and vitamin B, is helpful.

Treatment of underlying medical conditions like thyroid disease, anaemia, and hormonal imbalances may useful in prevention.

CHAPTER TEN
Final and Important Tips

If it is true now that you are in search of picking of treatment, you must be aware of a few points stated below.

1. It's quite normal to drop near about one hundred fifty tress of hair every day. Don't get horrified when you notice hair strand creping around your shoulder and also on the floor. What you need is hair loss treatment with right Hair care products.

2. Avoid combing hair when wet because they're vulnerable to falling or breaking. Use a broad-teeth comb after drying your hair and always comb the hair from the top that is the root to the bottom of hair very tenderly.

3. Trimming hair in a regular interval is helpful for your hair. Cut those strands about 2 or 3 inches in every 6 – 8 weeks to prevent the rip ends to turn out again.

4. Never leave the labels of the hair product unread. For the last few years, lot of attention has been given on one of ingredients. It is sulphate in shampoos that is responsible for good and shiny hair. It is one of the important things of your Hair Care Products.

5. Never get your hair dyed if your hair is dry
    sort. However, if you can't resist that gorgeous
    shade of brown, especially under the winter
    sun then follow the expert advice.

6. Using of hair lightener is the best idea to make
    your health good. Use lemon, chamomile tea or
    best hair oil as they work as great hair
    lighteners. Also, you can apply lemon juice and
    can spray lemon over your hair.

    Also, you the infused chameleon tea and can
    wash your hair with infused chamomile tea. So,
    it is advisable to wash your hair with shampoo
    or include honey to the water for washing your
    hair.

    As hair expertise, I'm advising to stay away
    from hair color if your hair is too dry by nature,
    but if you can't resist yourself from coloring
    your hair, then you should use the right hair
    oil, chamomile tea or lemon, especially in
    winter for better health of your hair.

    In that case, just spray lemon juice mixed water
    over your head before going out of your
    home. In addition, you can use chamomile tea
    liquor as a hair conditioner. Add honey to the
    water which you use for washing your hair.

Though the hair needs taking care of with hair oil all through the year, winter is the time when hair lack nourishment due to climatic variation. Feel revitalized and hydrate your hair leaving it feeling awesome with right Natural Hair Care Products.

CHAPTER ELEVEN
20 Effective Ways to Stop Hair Loss in Men

- Treat dietary deficiencies

- Telogen effluvium

- Reduce alcoholic

- Avoid smoking

- Diet

- Medication: Rogaine (Minoxidil)

- Avoid brushing wet hair

- De-stress

- Biotin: Biotin, also known as vitamin H

- Hydration

- Avoid constant heating and drying

- Avoid Frequent hair coloring

- Sweat-free scalp

- Prevent traction alopecia

- Regular physical activity such as walking and swimming

- Treat itchy scalp on time

- Overactive thyroid gland or hypoactive thyroid gland are both known to cause hair loss.

- Increased sugars may increase the risk of folliculitis

- Alopecia causing medications

- Regular massaging of the scalp may increase blood circulation in the scalps and help you to relax and improve scalp health.